A Study on Human Perception

George K. Laopodis

March 2019

Contents

PROLOGUE

What if I told you that the world, out there, the one we all experience is not real? It does not exist.

What if I told you there are no colors or sounds, no taste or smell out there? Do you think that our reality, around us, is occurring exactly this moment, right now? Like it or not, none of these statements are true. There is no color or sound, there is no smell or taste.

Our brain is "feeding" us this wonderful *construct* of a delightful world so we can survive this earth's environment.

To see the *real world* as it is, we would have to be different beings to accommodate the sensors that are *required* to perceive *everything* that is going on out there. Even then, no colors no sounds, and so on.

Not only that, but the proposition that our world is occurring exactly right now is also not true. The construct of the world we experience is always in the *past*. *Life, out there, is not real and it's not right now.*

Not only this is true on a biological level, a level that we are going to examine, but at a philosophical level of existence, a level that we are also going to examine.

It's not enough that the world out there is colorless and soundless and does not exist and it's not occurring right now, the *construct* of the world that our brain is developing for us is very limited in its depth and we can only observe a small section of the "real".

Imagine yourself in a deep diver's suit, the one that has the metal round helmet and a window in the front. That is how we humans are observing the real world around us. The rest is made up by our brains. We only see and hear a very small part of the world, and even that, is not real or right now.

Here is a quick and cute example that will give a hint.

Have you noticed that our pets[1] "know" that someone is coming close to our front door, sometime *before* we hear

---

[1] Cats' frequency range goes up to 64 kHz, which is 1.6 octaves above the range of a human, and even 1 octave above the range of a dog. When listening for something, a cat's ears will swivel in that direction; Cats can judge within three inches (8 cm) the location of a sound being made one yard (1 m) away—this can be useful for locating their prey.

anything?   That is because their range of the acoustic frequency spectrum is wider than ours and they can hear higher frequencies that we are not able to hear.

What we must ascertain from this is that there is a real-world, out there, which is invisible to us. If our dogs and cats can hear it, it must exist.

Our brains are *making* our lives all up. To make matters more interesting, we cannot recognize this process all by ourselves. One has to be *shown*. The *real* world out there and the "real" world residing inside our brains are not identical or even the same.

Let us examine how this is possible.

George Laopodis

April, 2019

California, USA

A Biological Experiment with an Eye

Many years ago, I attended an ophthalmology college in Boston, Massachusetts. I was very young then and my educational goal was to become an optical professional working with geometric optics.

One of the requirements was a course called ophthalmic lab. It was a laboratory course designed to teach students like me the practical side of optical theory. I like to describe one specific day in that laboratory because it is *crucial* to our endeavor to understand human perception as related to our understanding of reality.

This particular laboratory session required that all students dissected donated eyes. *It is something I would never do now* but back then I was very young and the school required that I took part in that endeavor.

The eyes that were "donated" to the school for this purpose came from cows. Cows' eyes are very large and they are extremely similar to human eyes.

The purpose of the dissections was to experience personally the construction of the human eye and also to understand how light rays enter the eye and how it focuses on the retina in the back of the eye. In other words, we had to observe and learn the mechanism behind how a human perceives the world around them within the eye. I rather not get into the details of the dissection here but I would like to describe briefly the inner structure of the eye because it is *very important to us.*

Light enters the human eye in the front through a bi-convex lens[2]. This human lens is attached to the eye structure through a few muscles called *ocular* muscles and they are responsible for changing the thickness of the lens so it can accommodate images that are close to the subject or very far. For example, when a human being looks at something close to them these muscles change the lens to be very

---

[2] A biconvex lens collimates a beam of light passing through the lens converging to a spot (a focus) behind the lens. In this case, the lens is called a positive or converging lens. The distance from the lens to the spot is the focal length of the lens, which is commonly abbreviated f in diagrams and equations.

thick, and inversely, the lens becomes very thin when observing images very far.

These muscles then change the optical characteristics of the lens and its optical power depending on what one looks at and how far it is. It is all based on accepted optical mathematic theory.

The human lens does this to make sure that the objects we observe are always focused perfectly on the central retina (it's called *fovea centralis*) at the back of the eye. As you can ascertain from graph 2, the *cones* of the retina are used for color vision, and the rods of the retina for darker images (black and white images during a night with no light).

Please note the "blind spot" a few degrees from the fovea in graph 3 that is caused by the existence of the optical nerve connection that has no rods or cones. This little detail has enormous repercussions in our human perception of the real world.

Now that we are familiar with the construction of the human eye let us continue with the results of my dissection of the eye that I mentioned earlier.

The eye is filled with a transparent jelly-like substance called *aqueous humour* and that is what is gives the eye its round shape. When the eye is pierced with a surgical knife the humour escapes and the eye collapses.

Further dissection revealed the lens and the retina in the back of the eye (the retina looks like a bluish, and wet multispectral reflecting film). Since the eye had collapsed because of the absence of the humour, one has to manually *reconstruct* the eye to discover how it works when light enters it.

Finally, I did manage to reconstruct the eye under my observation and I set it up in such a way as to have a *light source* and an *object* form an *image* (of the object) at the back of the eye at the retina. It worked perfectly. One could observe a smaller image at the retina, perfectly formed. But t*here was a small issue with the image...*

As you can ascertain from figure 5, the image of the object at the back of the eye was *inverted*.

The image of the object was upside down but consistent with the mathematics involved[3].

This small detail did not surprise me, mathematically speaking, but at the time I failed to understand the meaning of this detail as it relates to human perception. It took me several years before I understood the implications of this small detail and the other detail concerning the blind spot of graph 3.

Let us address one more feature of the eye because it will help us understand *all* the real world out there, one that we will never experience directly; that is the sensitivity *range* of the human eye as related to the electrometric spectrum.

$$\frac{1}{f} = (n-1)\left[\frac{1}{R_1} - \frac{1}{R_2} + \frac{(n-1)d}{nR_1R_2}\right],$$

[3] Lensmaker's equation. (f=focal length of the lens, n=index of refraction of the lens, R1 and R2=Radii of the two sides of the lens and d=thickness of the lens)

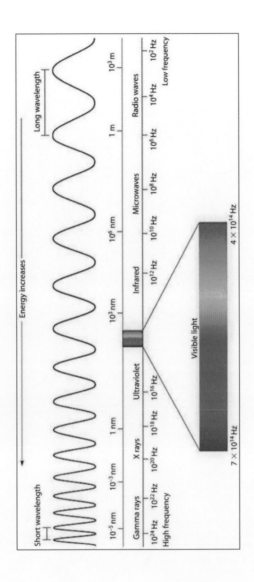

Figure 1 The entire electromagnetic spectrum is much more than just visible light. It encompasses of range of wavelengths of energy that our human eyes can't see. (Courtesy of miniphysics.com)

As one can deduce from fig. 1, we can only optically observe a very small part of the real world as it exists out there. Can one imagine what the real world looks like out there if our eyes were sensitive to the whole electromagnetic spectrum? Can one imagine a world where one could hear the whole acoustic spectrum?

The brain is "shielding" us from all that by using our memory (patterns) and some new data streams from all its sensors to create an illusionary world that does not exist. And the best part is that we *all* think it is real.

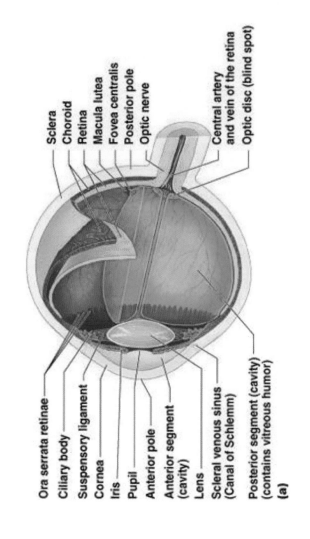

Sclera
Choroid
Retina
Macula lutea
Fovea centralis
Posterior pole
Optic nerve

Central artery
and vein of the retina
Optic disc (blind spot)

Ora serrata retinae
Ciliary body
Suspensory ligament
Cornea
Iris
Pupil
Anterior pole
Anterior segment
(cavity)
Lens
Scleral venous sinus
(Canal of Schlemm)
Posterior segment (cavity)
(contains vitreous humor)
(a)

Figure 2 Human eye anatomy

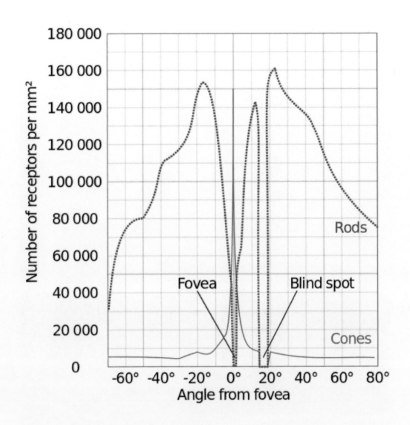

Figure 3 Photoreceptor distribution in the retina (rods and cones[4]) Courtesy of Cmglee @ commons.wikimedia.org

---

[4] A photoreceptor cell is a specialized type of neuroepithelial cell found in the retina that is capable of visual phototransduction. The great biological importance of photoreceptors is that they convert light into signals that can stimulate biological processes. To be more specific, photoreceptor proteins in the cell absorb photons, triggering a change in the cell's membrane potential using Vitamin A.

There are currently three known types of photoreceptor cells in mammalian eyes: rods, cones, and intrinsically photosensitive retinal ganglion cells. The two classic photoreceptor cells are rods and cones, each contributing information used by the visual system to form a representation of the visual world, sight. The rods are narrower than the cones and distributed differently across the retina, but the chemical process in each that supports phototransduction is similar. A third class of mammalian photoreceptor cell was discovered during the 1990s: the intrinsically photosensitive retinal ganglion cells. These cells do not contribute to sight directly, but are thought to support circadian rhythms and pupillary reflex.

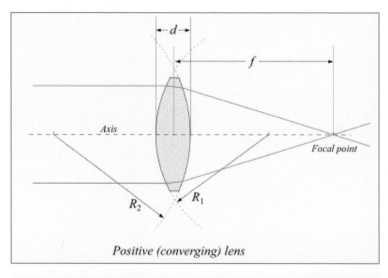

Positive (converging) lens

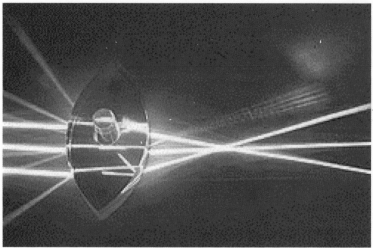

Figure 4 A Bi-convex lens similar to a human lens converging to a single focus at the focal point. (courtesy of Wikipedia.com)

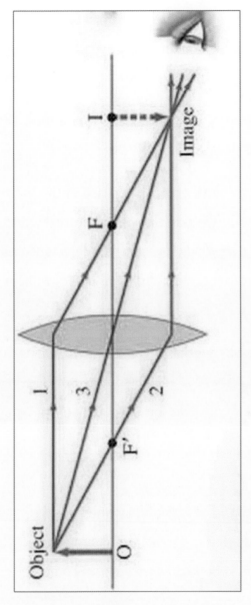

Figure 5 Formation of an inverted image through a human lens using light rays (Courtesy of amherst.edu)

A few years later, those two small details will eventually begin to trouble and affect my perception of reality as I am about to do to your perception of reality right now.

It is deceivingly simple really; The question that started disturbing me was as this:

If the image of an object is focused in the retina inverted how is it that we don't perceive the real-world *inverted*? That is, if everything we observe (objects) comes through the eyes to the optical nerve *upside-down*, how come the world I observe is right-side up?

And there was another such detail that had me puzzled and confused; if there is a blind spot near the fovea, how is it that we don't observe such a spot in our everyday vision?

I finally realized that there can be only one explanation to this dilemma; Our brain must be *manipulating* our perception of reality and the world about us. I was forced to conclude that my "real" world, around me, was not *real* but an almost perfect *construct* of my brain.

That's just great. I am observing a world around me that is a *creation* of my brain, not the *real* world.

It looks like a "real" world (the brain forms our world based on a few real-world data updates and memory patterns of our surroundings) but it is not *real*; it is an *imaginary* construct of our brain.

That is why we don't observe the world upside down or the blind spot in our retina; our brain "filters" those details out and reconstructs the images to provide a "normal" world image.

And there was something else that finally convinced me of this whole mechanism. Light is extremely fast[5] but it not *instantaneous*. Light takes time to propagate from one point to another. For example, it takes light about 1.3 seconds to travel from the moon to the earth.

You obviously can see where I am going with this. If light rays take some small time to reflect off the object I am observing then travel through my eyes, to my optical nerve, and finally to my brain to be analyzed and interpreted, then whatever I observe as *real* is not the present but the past. By the time our brain analyzes all the incoming signals and forms the world for us, the original image could be gone or

---

[5] 299,792,458 meters/second or about 186,000 miles/second in vacuum.

changed. We always observe the world around us a little late; we are always experiencing and live a little in the *past*.

So, we live our entire lives immersed in a reconstruction of the real world *thinking* that the world we observe is real and is occurring right now.

Not only do we observe a *construct* of the world about us on a biological and physical level, but we also experience the world as a *"construct"* on a philosophical level.

And this is where we are going next. Let us examine our "real" world about us in *philosophical terms*.

We, the Cave Dwellers

In 1999, the *Wachowski "Brothers"* (Lana and Lilly Wachowski), released an enormously successful movie called *The Matrix* starring Keanu Reeves, Laurence Fishburne, Carrie-Anne Moss, and others. To date, this movie has won 4 Oscars (37 wins and 49 nominations) and has grossed close to half a billion dollars. It is one of my favorite films and I suggest that you should watch it.

The graphics of this movie were exceptional as was the acting by all the participants. But what made this movie so unique, remarkable, and unforgettable was the story. The story of a man called Mr. Anderson.

If you have seen the movie, that's great. If not, I will briefly describe the story in the next few paragraphs because it is extremely important to our present study on human perception and reality.

Even though the Matrix story is so unique and remarkable, one cannot say that it is new.

The elementary story in the movie Matrix is about 2400 years old and first originate and was developed by the Greek philosopher Plato[6] in his little publication called *Republic[7] (book VII).*

Let us agree to spend some time on the story of Mr. Anderson in the film Matrix.

---

[6] Plato (427-347 BC) was an Athenian philosopher during the Classical period in Ancient Greece, founder of the Platonist school of thought, and the Academy, the first institution of higher learning in the Western world. He is widely considered the pivotal figure in the history of Ancient Greek and Western philosophy, along with his teacher, Socrates, and his most famous student, Aristotle. Plato has also often been cited as one of the founders of Western political philosophy, religion and spirituality. The so-called Neoplatonism of philosophers like Plotinus and Porphyry influenced Saint Augustine and thus Christianity. Alfred North Whitehead once noted: "the safest general characterization of the European philosophical tradition is that it consists of a series of footnotes to Plato."

[7] The Republic is a Socratic dialogue, written by Plato around 380 BC, concerning justice (δικαιοσύνη), the education of the young, the order and character of the just city-state, and the just man. It is Plato's best-known work, and has proven to be one of the world's most influential works of philosophy and political theory, both intellectually and historically.

In the dialogue, Socrates discusses with various Athenians and foreigners the meaning of justice and whether the just man is happier than the unjust man. They consider the natures of existing regimes and then propose a series of different, hypothetical cities in comparison, culminating in Kallipolis, a city-state ruled by a philosopher king. They also discuss the theory of forms, the immortality of the soul, and the role of the philosopher and of poetry in society. The dialogue's setting seems to be during the Peloponnesian War.

Mr. Thomas Anderson is a young man who lives in a big American city working as a computer programmer for a very large corporation like Microsoft or Google.

Mr. Anderson's life appears to be normal and content and although he seems to be an exceptional programmer, he is not a very consistent employee and he has problems with his manager.

Unknown to his manager, Mr. Anderson has another very secret life. He is also a famous computer *hacker*[8] going by the *handle Neo*.

Neo appears content with his life but he is also a man searching for something. He is not sure what he is looking for but it is obvious that something is missing from his life and he is searching online for it even though he is not exactly sure what he is looking for.

So, Neo hopes that another famous computer *hacker* called *Morpheus* may hold the answers to his quest.

---

[8] A computer hacker is any skilled computer expert that uses their technical knowledge to overcome a problem. While "hacker" can refer to any skilled computer programmer, the term has become associated in popular culture with a "security hacker", someone who, with their technical knowledge, uses bugs or exploits to break into computer systems.

Morpheus, however, is very elusive and not an easy man to find. That is until this certain night when Neo receives a cryptic computer message from him. Morpheus wants to meet Neo.

During a very rainy night in this music club, Neo encounters another famous young hacker called *Trinity* who finally takes Neo to meet Morpheus in this lofty abandoned building. Morpheus communicates to Neo that he knows what Neo has been looking for and he is prepared to share the information with him but there is *one condition*.

Morpheus cannot communicate to Neo what he wants to know; he can only *show* him. And for that to occur, Neo has to swallow a red pill so Morpheus can *find* Neo's body and free him! Morpheus also *mentions* that if Neo takes the red pill, there is no going back for Neo. The process is *irreversible*.

I am certain that at this point Neo is not only intrigued and perplexed but also extremely skeptical because he doesn't understand what Morpheus means by finding his (Neo's) body, Neo is standing right in front of Morpheus, his body is right there. Neo must have felt like *Alice sliding down into the rabbit hole, with all possible haste.*

Neo finally decides he wants to know what this is all about and he swallows the red pill.

The red pill is a small computer program that will pinpoint the location of Neo's body and also it disrupts his connections with the *Matrix.*

The next part of the film that shows where Neo's body exists is dismal, to say the least. Neo's body is enclosed in this transparent "shell" full of thick liquid that looks like a coffin. This *pod* is attached to this round tall tower, one of thousand such pod attachments among hundreds of such towers! There were millions of these pods in this huge chamber.

The red pill[9] causes the liquid in Neo's pod to drain out and Neo is brought out of his *suspended animation* while all the hose attachments to his body fall off, one by one.

---

[9] There was a choice. There was a blue pill also that would have left Neo sleeping back at his apartment.

Neo sits up and looks around to see all the towers full of pods with people in them. (fig. 6)

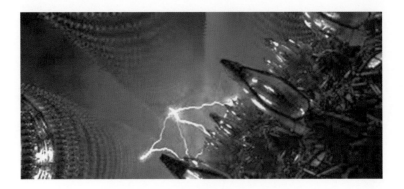

Figure 6 Fetus fields in Matrix

Suddenly, a port opens in Neo's pod and he slides out of the pod and down to this pool of water where he is caught by a mechanical hand and brought aboard a hovercraft called *Nebuchadnezzar*[10].

---

[10] Nebuchadnezzar II ("O god Nabu, preserve/defend my firstborn son"), king of Babylon c. 605 BC – c. 562 BC, was the longest-reigning and most powerful monarch of the Neo-Babylonian Empire.

His father Nabopolassar was an official of the Neo-Assyrian Empire who rebelled in 620 BC and established himself as the king of Babylon. Nebuchadnezzar ascended the throne in 605 BC and subsequently fought several campaigns in the West, where Egypt was trying to organize a coalition against him. His conquest of Judah is described in the Bible's Books of Kings and Book of Jeremiah. His capital, Babylon, is the largest archaeological site in the Middle East.

The Bible remembers him as the destroyer of Solomon's Temple and the initiator of the Babylonian captivity. He is an important character in the Book of Daniel, a collection of legendary tales and visions dating from the 2nd century BC.

Neo finally wakes up on this ship and he meets the *real* Morpheus (the captain) and his crew including Trinity.

But you thought that Neo and Morpheus met and were having a conversation in this *tall building* during a very *rainy night*? Why was Neo in a pod and Morpheus in a ship? This is going to get a little complicated at this point but persevere. There is a logical explanation.

The tall building, the rainy night, and Neo's life and city are not real. There are constructs (powerful programs) of a very powerful computer that are *fed* to Neo's and everyone else's brain to make them believe that they live a normal life, in a normal city, while they are all in pods, slumbering their life away and providing the machines with their body thermal energy[11] to power it and all its computers. From their birth until their death.

Once Neo started to recuperate from his life-long slumber and his body started to overcome the atrophy of all his muscles, it was time to hear the rest of the story from Morpheus.

---

[11] For a typical human sleeping the rate is about 13 Btu/h or 4.2 Watts.

Morpheus had a remarkable story for Neo. It was rather shocking actually.

Many years ago, the people of the earth had succeeded in developing artificial intelligence (AI) in machines to a very high degree of perfection. The AI was so successful that humans allowed the new intelligent machines to run most of the world for them, freeing humans to do other things. They even trusted the machines with the defense of the kingdom.

But the humans had made the machines so perfect and so intelligent that the machines started to take full control of all human life on earth including control of the humans themselves. Understandably, that situation was unacceptable to the human race, so they started a great big war against the AI machines to take back control.

The war against the AI was brutal, to say the least, because machines never give up until their computer directives are realized to the full. The war continued for many years and it appeared that the machines were starting to win this war. The humans were very desperate and decided to do something extremely drastic.

Since the AI machines were powered mainly by the sun (solar radiation energy), the humans decided to *stop* the sun from radiating energy!

The humans succeeded with their sun shut-down project but there were chaotic repercussions. The earth became barren and started dying. Life on earth started dying also as did the cities and everything else. People could no longer live on the surface of the earth and moved deep inside it.

This is when Morpheus showed Neo a visual of what earth looked like at the present. The images were so cataclysmic that Neo had a near collapse. He just could not believe what Morpheus was telling him.

The earth looked like an enormous atom bomb had wiped everything on it almost to the ground. And that was not all. The worst of the story was to come next.

But the machines were not stopped as hoped. The AI switched its power source just in time to save itself from destruction. It switched from solar energy to battery power. Where did they find such enormous energy from batteries?

By slaving the humans from birth to death in pods to harness their thermal radiation. They had turned a human being into a battery.

On top of all this, the AI also created a construct (a computer program) that imitated real-life to almost perfection and they fed this program to all the humans in their pods through a physical link to their brain.

This alternate artificial reality was called *The Matrix*.

The humans in captivity never knew that they were captive and used. They were very happy with their AI life. They could not tell the difference. For example, Neo could have spent his whole life in a pod thinking he was a computer programmer working for a large software company.

But all was not lost for the human race. One man somehow woke up in a pod and freed himself. He then started to free other people so that they created a new city for themselves, deep inside the earth, free from the AI. The city was called *Zion*. And that is how Morpheus and his crew came to be.

Neo could never go back now. He was out of the Matrix for good…like it or not he was *free*.

Morpheus also explained to Neo that he was freed because an oracle had prophesized that Neo would save the human race. Neo must save the world.

I will not go any further with the Matrix story, it is not important to our research in human perception of reality or I should say the *illusion of reality*? Feel free to watch the film.

As I mentioned earlier, the story I just described to you is not new.

Plato was the first to consider this particular perception of reality and I like to describe to you what Plato philosophized. As you will ascertain shortly, our perception of the real world and life *is not as real* as we all think.

So, let me summarize what the film Matrix is suggesting.

Neo, a computer programmer for a large corporation that resides in a very large American city believes that what he sees and feels are real. Unfortunately, the reality is that Neo is in a pod, in a comma, supplying body thermal energy to power a big machine that has taken over the earth. To make matters more interesting, Neo is "fed" a construct of real-life through a cable attached and connected to the back of his brain by "the machine". This "imprisonment" is imperceptible to Neo. Neo thinks he lives in a city and works for a company as a programmer.

I just described briefly, the main theme of the film Matrix. But as you know, I also just described Plato's philosophical idea concerning the education of young people in the city of Athens around 340 BC. The two concepts are almost identical as we will discover next.

Plato, in Book VII of the *Republic,* introduces his idea concerning reality with a very interesting example that is very helpful in understanding the concept he is proposing.

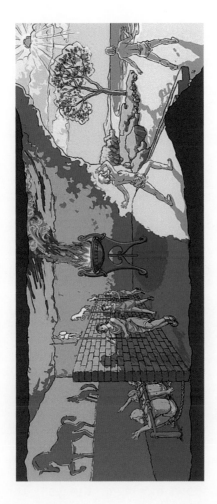

Figure 7 Plato's Cave[12] (Courtesy of 4edges)

I would like to present to you Plato's *allegory of the cave* which introduces his philosophical awareness of the *illusion of reality*.

The only correction I want to make to the illustration of the cave in fig. 7 is this: the cave is carved rather deeper in the earth that the image shows. One has to ascend many steps to exit; it is not at the same level as the prisoners.

So, there is a cave (see fig 7), deep in the ground and there is a wall in the middle of the cave. On one side of this long wall, there are prisoners (think of Neo's situation) that are all tied up to one side of the wall *all their life*. They are tied to the wall in such a way that these prisoners can only see what is in front of them and nothing else.

Everything the prisoners can observe in front of them are these dark shadows moving on the wall. They see various things like the shadow of a horse and the shadow of a soldier and shadows of dogs or wolves moving in front of them.

What these prisoners do not know or realize is that behind the wall they are tied to are various people holding up and moving all these statues on long poles.

These people are holding up these statues of things like the statue of a horse and the statue of a soldier and statues of dogs or wolves. These "pole-holding" people are walking in this corridor from one side to the other.

Now, behind these pole people, there is a large fire on a pedestal that is casting shadows of the statues on the wall in front of the prisoners. These shadows of real things are *the reality of the prisoners*.

One fine day, one of the prisoners of the wall is *freed*. Please note that I did not *write* escaped. The correct word is freed because a prisoner cannot escape the wall *unless* someone (not a prisoner) liberates him. The reason for that is that the prisoners do not know they are prisoners and they don't realize that what they see on the wall in front of them are just shadows of the real things. This paragraph above provided the choice between the Red or the Blue pill for Neo in the film Matrix.

The prisoners simply do not know what is occurring behind the wall, so the shadows on the wall are reality to them.

The prisoner that is freed looks behind him for the first time in his life and sees the statues on the poles and the various people that are holding them.

He also observes the fire that is casting the shadows on the wall and realizes that everything he believed real was an illusion of reality. His whole life he believed in a world of shadows. He was utterly shocked. His real world was a real projection manipulated by some other people that he didn't even know were there.

This freed prisoner also realizes something about real knowledge. The human instinct is to observe and learn so the prisoners were convinced that the moving shadows on the wall offered them knowledge. For example, they perhaps started playing the game of shadows. They knew that if there was a soldier on the wall followed by a wolf, then the next image would be a horse. *"See? There is a soldier and a wolf, I bet the next image is a wolf."* They had "real knowledge".

The freed prisoner finally screams OMG...all I thought real were machinations of others.

Then suddenly, the freed prisoner notices something new; there is an exit to this cave high up there. There was light entering the door exit. The prisoner decided to reach for the exit but the way to the exit is rough.

The ascent is tiring and there were many steps to climb. But after a long hard journey, he finally arrives at the exit and steps outside. The prisoner sees real horses and real soldiers and the real sun and he again exclaims...OMG.

What he thought was real down there were just shadows of the real things. These real things are also much more vivid and beautiful to him. The sun was also really bright unlike the glow of the fire in the cave.

Now that we have examined the cave and the search for a higher level of truth and reality, let us examine the contents of the cave in a much more detailed manner.

Who do the prisoners represent? They represent us, you and I, all of us, all the people on earth. We are born prisoners and we stay in that prison for the rest of our lives.

We all begin with ignorance chained to our perceived shadow reality. I am afraid this is how it is. We are all born only knowing the walls around us and the life that we grow up with. We don't know anything else. We are trapped in our present condition…forever. The shadows on the wall are our reality and the cave is a symbol of our ignorance of that reality.

Now let us turn our attention to the people behind the wall, the ones that hold the statues, the shadow theater puppeteers. Who are these puppeteers, these manipulators of our reality on the wall for their benefit? Who has vested interests to manipulate our reality?

- Family
- Friends
- Marketers
- Media
- Politicians
- Government
- Religion
- Schools

Now, even though these people manipulate our reality for their benefit and are a bit more aware than the general public, they still live in the cave of ignorance, just like us. There is no escaping the cave of ignorance. One can only be freed from the cave *by someone else*!

Now let us focus our attention on the many steps that lead to the outside of the cave. As I noted, the way to the exit of the cave is really steep, hard, and laborious. Only individuals with a strong belief in *the ideal* will succeed. The ascend to freedom of the cave is a metaphor toward a higher truth and the ideal life.

One has to have the courage to admit that perhaps the life they lived was not as *real* as they thought. We should perhaps change the way we perceive life in general. That is why the steps to freedom are so hard to climb. It requires a complete change of perception.

To make matters more difficult for the prisoners of the cave, the ascend to the highest level of enlightenment becomes much more difficult if you are an older person.

At one point in the film Matrix, Neo almost had a heart attack after he realized what his real-world looked like.

Morpheus tried to explain to Neo the reason behind the difficulty of accepting reality as it is. Morpheus explained that "they don't usually free older people. They only free people at a very young age. These youngsters are much more likely to accept the new reality because they have not been in *stasis* for very long and therefore, they are more open to change. Neo was an exception."

As you remember, I mentioned earlier that prisoners cannot escape the cave by themselves, they had to be freed by someone else. So how is it that the freed prisoner we discussed earlier made it to the surface? How was he freed?

Someone came down the cave and freed him.

The reason for that is that most of us are complacent. We are content and happy with the way we are currently and we do not object to our way of life. Just like Neo, we are gratified with our present situation. Radical change requires a very strong effort and it's a long and winding road to freedom. Most people will resist this new vision... *"just go away and leave me alone."*

I am sure Neo had second thoughts after he was freed concerning the "red pill" he swallowed.

Perhaps he should have chosen the "blue pill" that would have left him in his illusionary but comfortable world.

What other situations can wake us up to reality and break our chains from the wall in the cave?

One way is a severe illness. When we get deathly sick and we make it out alive, is one way to wake up. After such trauma, we perceive life and the world in a very different manner, as it is. We realize that there is no security, we are not safe and life is a very fragile thing that can break very easily at any time.

Another way to break the chains is by visiting and living in a foreign country that is contrary to the one we grew up in. Then one realizes that the manner that we grew up with is not the *only way* of life. There are other modes of life out there that are foreign to us.

One more technique to break the chains is participating in higher education where you are exposed to ideas that you never heard of.

Education can force us to reconsider everything we grew up with. What we learned in high school pale by comparison to the exposition of higher education. This is the reason behind the idea that *all* citizens should be philosophers.

We must understand that most people will not turn off their TV just to read Sartre's *Being and Nothingness*. Someone has to force them to do that.

So, let us return briefly to Plato's cave of complacency and the prisoners within. Let's assume that the freed prisoner that made it to the outside of the cave suddenly remembered his fellow prisoners in the cave still chained to the wall and decides to do something about it. He wants to tell his friends down there of his new reality and the illusion of the shadows they are experiencing.

I am certain that the first sentence out of their mouth would be *"are you crazy?"* His fellow prisoners have a good comfortable life there and they have real knowledge. For example, they know what shadow comes after they see a horse and a soldier. They just don't want to hear him. The way to cognitive freedom is paved with thorns.

Before we move on to our next chapter, I like to remind you why we were addressing Plato's allegory of the cave. I was trying to advocate that human perception cannot be trusted to provide us with the real world on a *philosophical level*.

We will transfer now and examine our perception of reality as it is presented to us by our brain at a *biological level*.

Do you think that the wonderful colors we perceive around us, the sounds we hear, and the smells of real life are out there? Do you think that all your sensory perceptions out there exist in your city somewhere? They do not. They only exist in our brains. Let examine then how this is possible.

The Human Brain

I have worked in astronomy most of my life and I like to tell you that the universe is the most complex entity that exists (without humans). I cannot. The most intricate entity in this world is a three-pound object in our cranium and it's called the *brain*.

Everything we feel and hold dear, our hopes and disappointments, all that we care about including reality and memory exist in there.

Do you think reality, as you perceive it in your everyday life, is real? Do you think that what you smell and taste are real? They are not, reality is an illusion created by your brain.

Let's return to the example we addressed briefly in the prologue.

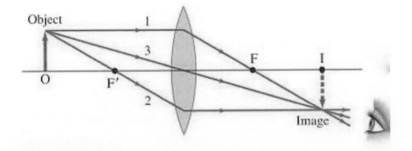

Figure 8 The Inverted Object

As I mentioned earlier, within the human eye the objects we see arrive at the retina inverted. (see fig. 8). This inversion is based on an optical formula we also examined. If the image of the object arriving at the retina is inverted, how is it that our real world is not inverted? The only answer to this question is that the brain is creating our reality...continuously.

There is no way out of this conclusion. Like it or not our brain is *feeding* us an excellent imitation of the real world. If we could somehow see the real world as it exists, out there, it would be very *frightening* and *overwhelming*.

No colors, no sounds, smells or tastes, and so on. Our brains invent all that for us.

Let us examine in detail how the brain accomplishes this amazing presentation and why it looks just like reality.

Our reality has much *less* to do with what is occurring out there and much *more* with what is happening *inside* our brain.

Let examine one member of our sensory mechanisms as an example. It is the most complicated of all our sensors; the optical system.

As I mentioned, an object out there reflects light rays to our eyes. The rays reflected off the object travel through our eye lenses get inverted and arrive (*converges*) as such on the retina. At the retina, with the help of Vitamin A (it's called *retinol*), our rods or cones convert Vitamin A to an electrical signal by a chemoelectrical process.

This is a very delicate conversion because when the light hits retinol, retinol decomposes and has to be replenished immediately, or else we could not go seeing[13].

---

[13] So, make sure you take enough Vitamin A

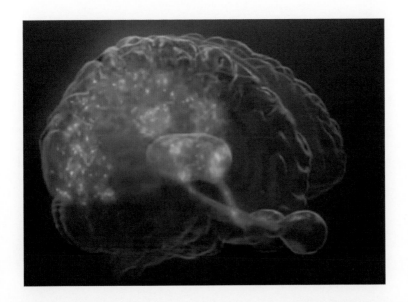

Figure 9 Image of the thalamus and visual cortex (courtesy of BBC)

The optical wavelengths of the rays entering our eyes are converted to electrical signals and travel through our optical nerve connections to the *thalamus* where they are examined there for use (see fig 9).

From there, the electrical signals travel again and end up at the *visual cortex,* at the back of the brain. A healthy human optical system, as a whole, uses about 30 percent of the brain's space. One must imagine the enormous amount of data entering our eyes every minute.

All this huge stream of *electrical signals* moving from the thalamus to the visual cortex, all the time, continuously.

It should be noted that what we all perceive as colors, sounds, scents, are different wavelengths of light, acoustic compressions of the air converted to electrical signals, and the complicated chemical analysis results from our smells.

One would think that the return stream to the thalamus from the visual cortex would be equal or smaller.

The return stream of signals (the traffic) is almost 500 percent bigger than the upstream. Our visual cortex is simply providing much more data back to the thalamus that it receives!

Let's examine specifically what data the brain uses to make such an elaborate construct for our benefit. There are two main streams of data that the brain uses to form the world for us.

I. One stream of data originates in our memory patterns regarding our surroundings, saved in our brains over time since we were born.

II.   The other stream of data comes from all the sensors that the brain is attached to (like the eyes, skin, nose, and ear... in real-time).

Based mostly on the memory patterns of our surroundings in our brains and *some real-time* data, the brain creates a world that is remarkably real.   It would be too slow to create a new world every second just based on real streams of data. The brain would overload. It is insufficient because this mode is going to slow your thinking and you down to a crawl.

Instead, the brain uses our memories to construct our basic world[14] (which is almost instantaneous) and then it just updates the world with real data from our sensors as needed *only*.

I believe a better term for the *internal model* is the *best-fit (internal) model*. This is because each model must accommodate its particular environment perfectly and must have the ability to reset all such models and create a new one if necessary.

---

[14] It is called the *Internal Model*

We must remember that our brain sits isolated in our craniums, in total darkness making no sound. Our brains have never been exposed to the real world, out there. The brain is just an isolated, in the dark, super biological *interconnect* and it functions by using billions of *biological* capacitors, charging, and discharging as needed. These are the electronic signals the brain utilizes to communicate and exist.

We have more than seven billion people on this earth and they each have their unique *best-fit model*. Our brains have some similarities but we are all unique because our perspective of the world is based on our *internal model* which is unique for everyone on earth. Remember that reality is a *show* the brain is playing for us, in real-time, *continuously*.

Remember the diver's helmet that I mentioned earlier on page four? It is time to remove it and observe the rest of the real world that we have never seen before.

Humans can't see the whole range of the electromagnetic spectrum. If we did, we would not look like humans anymore.

The spectrum of wavelengths begins at below human acoustic levels and ends up in the region of gamma rays and beyond. We humans can only perceive only a very small percentage of the world *out there*.

The real world is colorless and odorless. The brain has made all that up through evolution and we just attach labels to them. The labels are there so we can communicate, they don't mean anything at all.

Only rays of light exist, reflecting everywhere, different chemicals in the air mixed with oxygen and a plethora of other rays, (like x-rays or cosmic rays and the others) flying everywhere around you and through you. If there was a way to see the real world as it is, I am not sure one would want to live in it. It will be too overwhelming.

As I mentioned, although we humans cannot see most of the world out there, there are ways to visualize how the real world appears *if* we could see it all. As you know, visually we can only see in a very small section of the whole spectrum that exists out there.

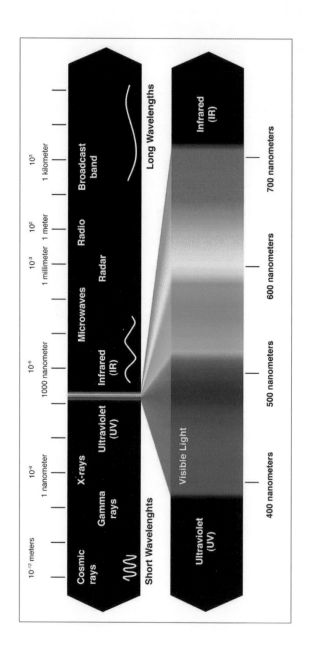

Figure 10 Most of the rest of the existing spectrum

For us humans, our possible visual range is between about 400nm = λ and 700nm = λ (λ=wavelength). the rest ninety-five percent of the world is simply not detected. The following images will provide a good idea of what "out there" really looks like.

We will start at the low end of the spectrum and the acoustic range of frequencies that exist out there. Only a small section of this acoustic spectrum is accessible to humans but -as you will observe- most of it is not. This is what we can hear in terms of acoustic waves through the air (space has no sound):

Our acoustic abilities (frequency range) are between about 20 Hz (λ/sec) and 40000 Hz while our furry friends can hear wavelengths up to 65000 Hz. Below that range and above it, we simply cannot hear a thing but the wavelengths are all there been emitted. See fig. 10 and 11.

Figure 12 shows how our real earth environment sounds like, although we cannot hear it. If we could hear at these frequencies then we could distinguish frequencies coming not only from our area but from the planets and the sun "hitting" the earth with frequencies all the time.

At the same time, you would be also be inundated continuously with *human*-made radar waves along with *space* made radar wavelengths bouncing off everything about you.

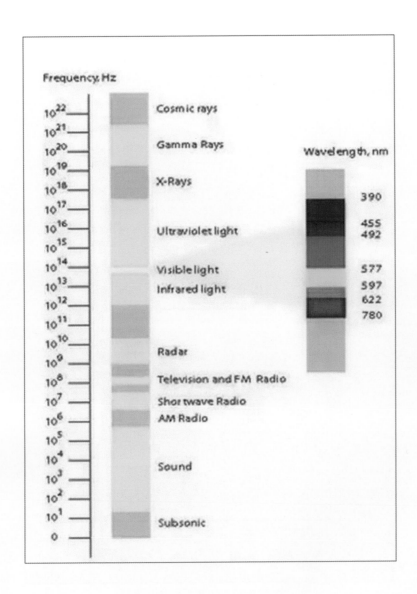

Figure 11 All Known frequencies[15]

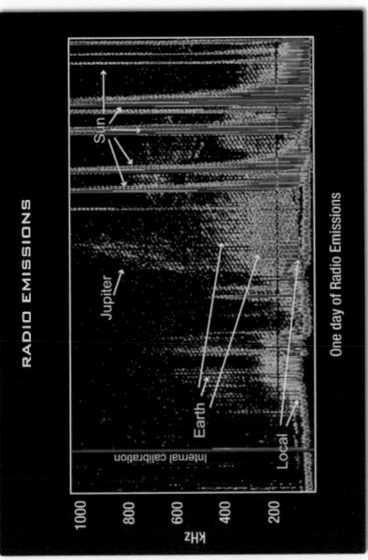

Figure 12 Acoustics from Space

Now that we addressed the acoustic spectrum and how it would sound to us if we could hear all of it, let us turn and examine how the visible and invisible spectrum would appear to us...if we could see it.

Please refer to figure 10. Not only we would be able to observe the sun rays as we do now but all the rays that we normally cannot detect.

Can one imagine if we all could see all the radiation about us? It would be overwhelming, awe-inspiring, and devastating.

Where can I start with the different radiation bombarding the earth from space? We have cosmic rays[16]. Cosmic rays have frequencies of oscillation in the upper exahertz region ($3x10^{19}$Hz to over $3x10^{27}$Hz). The wavelength(s) in this region of the spectrum are in the 0.050 to 0.001 nm range.

---

[16] Cosmic rays are a form of high-energy radiation, mainly originating outside the Solar System and even from distant galaxies. Upon impact with the Earth's atmosphere, cosmic rays can produce showers of secondary particles that sometimes reach the surface. Composed primarily of high-energy protons and atomic nuclei, they are originated either from the sun or from outside of our solar system. Data from the Fermi Space Telescope (2013) have been interpreted as evidence that a significant fraction of primary cosmic rays originates from the supernova explosions of stars. Active galactic nuclei also appear to produce cosmic rays, based on observations of neutrinos and gamma rays from blazar TXS 0506+056 in 2018

There is no way for our eyes to see these rays and if we could the question is *would you want to*?

That is not all, there is more.

Next, we have Gamma rays[17] raining down and coming up entering everything. These rays are in the range above 10 exahertz (less than 10^{19} Hz so their wavelength is in the region of 10 picometers.

"The natural outdoor exposure in the United Kingdom ranges from 0.1 to 0.5 µSv/h with a significant increase around known nuclear and contaminated sites. Natural exposure to gamma rays is about 1 to 2 mSv per year, and the average total amount of radiation received in one year per inhabitant in the USA is 3.6 mSv. There is a small

---

[17] Gamma ray or gamma radiation (symbol γ), is a penetrating electromagnetic radiation arising from the radioactive decay of atomic nuclei. It consists of the shortest wavelength electromagnetic waves and so imparts the highest photon energy. Paul Villard, a French chemist and physicist, discovered gamma radiation in 1900 while studying radiation emitted by radium. In 1903, Ernest Rutherford named this radiation gamma rays based on their relatively strong penetration of matter; he had previously discovered two less penetrating types of decay radiation, which he named alpha rays and beta rays in ascending order of penetrating power.
For low-dose exposure, for example among nuclear workers, who receive an average yearly radiation dose of 19 mSv, the risk of dying from cancer (excluding leukemia) increases by 2 percent. For a dose of 100 mSv, the risk increase is 10 percent. By comparison, risk of dying from cancer was increased by 32 percent for the survivors of the atomic bombing of Hiroshima and Nagasaki.

increase in the dose, due to naturally occurring gamma radiation, around small particles of high atomic number materials in the human body caused by the photoelectric effect."

If humans could see these rays perhaps, they could see the interaction that occurs when these rays enter the molecular structure of their own body.

So, let us add gamma rays to our *repertoire* of our imaginary capable everyday vision; we see cosmic rays, we see gamma rays, we see sun rays, what else can we see?

Let us not forget what comes next, x-rays. Let us imagine that we could see x-rays. (Superman can see (perhaps) x-rays but emitting x-rays with his eyes, is another thing altogether). If we could see x-rays life would be unbearable. Have you seen the movie *"Man with the X-Ray Eyes"*[18] (1963) with Ray Milland?

---

[18] Ray Milland plays Dr. James Xavier a brilliant scientist who understands that the human eye only perceives a tenth of the entire visual spectrum. Through his experiments he develops an eye drop that allows a monkey to see through hard material and his gal-pal Dr. Diane Fairfax (Diana Van der Vlis) is astounded at the discovery. Xavier turns to his friend Dr. Sam Brant (Harold J. Stone) to aid him in administering the drug on himself to record the details first hand, but Brant doesn't want to because too much is still unknown about the drug. Xavier goes forward with his plans and discovers a wealth of new visual abilities he

The man could see through everything including his girlfriend...very romantic. If we could see x-rays, theoretically, we could see the destruction of our body's DNA sequences as x-rays interact with them. I am not certain I would like to be capable of "seeing" x-rays.

Next, on the spectrum scale are Ultraviolet rays. Our optical sensors are not sensitive at this frequency range either so we cannot see them. Perhaps these rays have introduced themselves to you when you were sunbathing on the beach. These wavelengths are between 10 and 400 nm and frequencies between 8×10^{14} and 3×10^{16} (/per second). Blacklight is a certain frequency in the ultraviolet spectrum[19].

---

didn't possess before. His ability to see through material prevents a miss-diagnosed surgery but puts him at odds with the attending physician at his hospital. Brant tries to prevent Xavier from continuing the drug because of the physical damage to his system. In the midst of an argument Xavier accidentally causes the death of Brant and Diane convinces Xavier to flee until he can pull himself together and explain what happened. Xavier drops out of sight until Diane tracks him down and discovers that by continually using the vision drug Xavier has developed a sensitivity that has caused shocking changes in the doctor's persona. As the police close in and crosses paths with a religious preacher the doctor takes some actions that have drastic aftereffects.

[19] In humans, excessive exposure to UV radiation can result in acute and chronic harmful effects on the eye's dioptric system and retina. The risk is elevated at high altitudes and people living in high latitude countries where snow covers the ground right into early summer and sun positions even at zenith are low, are particularly at risk. Skin, the circadian and immune systems can also be affected.

As you can ascertain there is a good reason why we do not perceive much of the real world out there. I don't think we would want to.

After ultraviolet rays are the "visible rays", and we all know what that appears like. This is the only part of the real world out there that has a true equivalent construct in the "real" world inside our brain. Finally, there are radar, tv, radio, sound waves, and subsonic frequencies.

And that is how the real world out there sounds and looks like if we could see it. As I inquired before, does one want to live in an earth environment that is so chaotic and abyssal?

Overexposure to UVB radiation not only can cause sunburn but also some forms of skin cancer. However, the degree of redness and eye irritation (which are largely not caused by UVA) do not predict the long-term effects of UV, although they do mirror the direct damage of DNA by ultraviolet.

No Color, No Sound, Smell, or Taste

As I mentioned at the beginning of this study, I promised to demonstrate that there are no colors or sounds, smells, or tastes *out there* in the real world. Please note that I did not say that is also true inside our brains. The "real" world in our brain is not the *real* world out there. The world in our brain is not necessarily the real world, the one we exist in.

We must make certain at this point that we differentiate and understand the difference between the real world out there outside our bodies and the *construct* of the "real world" residing in our brains. The former is real and the latter is not.

Let us consider as an example the color green. We all know what the color green looks like.

But we have to remember that the words color and green are creations of our brains, *not nature.* In nature, that is, in the world out there, there are no "colors" or "blue".

There, in the real world exist only frequencies and reflections of various radiations one of them being the frequency of the color blue: Wavelength ~450–495 nm and frequency ~670–610 THz. As you can ascertain, there are no colors in nature, just radiation of certain frequencies.

We "label" the frequency above to make it easy to communicate with each other. Can you imagine saying to someone *"I love the wavelength of your eyes?"* Not very romantic. Colors and their names are just *labels* of natural phenomena that are fully understood by science.

Now you want to know about the phrase *"there are no colors."* In nature, out there, there are no colors, only wavelengths of radiation. *Colors*, these labels, are a figment of our human imagination; they simply do not exist in the real world out there.

The same principles apply to smell and taste (chemical compositions of the air or some substance) and sound which are acoustic wavelengths that travel through the air to our ears to be analyzed and converted to electrical signals.

These electronic signals are then compared to our memory banks and if found there only then they "become" some certain *taste or smell, sound or image.* Our brain *only* "speaks" the language of electrical discharges, in the dark, in total silence never seen the real world outside.

As I promised, there are no colors, no sounds, no smells, or tastes out there in the real world.

Epilogue

Some final thoughts. Think of your brain (you) as the CEO of a very large and complex corporation (you).

We can do many things very well but there are things that we simply not good at.

For example, have you driven to work so many times and when you got there you forgot exactly how you got there? The reason for that is that *you* didn't drive to work. You let your *subconscious* do it for you.

Think of the *unconscious* as the hardware of your brain or a *Reparative Actions Processing Unit* (RAPU). They are excellent at doing repetitive tasks very fast. So, when you walk, for example, we let our RAPU hardware to do it simply because the computations to just "walk" are so complex.

These computations have to be executed immediately or else you *face plant*. Our brain's CEO is not very good at that all. Only the RAPU can do that.

Of course, when it comes to decisions like *how much you should pay for a car* is a decision that you, the CEO must make because you excel at that, the RAPU could not even consider the calculation.

Finally, the brain is our "gatekeeper" to the *real world out there* for us. Evolution created this standard operating procedure within our brain to ensure the progression of the human species. It is not the *real* world we are experiencing but it is a very good model of the real world within many limitations as we have examined previously.

One last question for you before I go:

Do you think that the book and the words you just finished reading are real?

Credits

Most of the footnotes are courtesy of Wikipedia.

Other books by George K. Laopodis

- The Man of Adolf Hitler (Vol II - 2019)
- The Women of Adolf Hitler (Vol I - 2017)
- The Forgotten Voice of Jesus (Vol I - 2013)
- The Forgotten Gods of Israel (Vol II -2014)
- The Telescope Makers (2014)
- The Smart Animal 2018

Printed in Great Britain
by Amazon

43826654R00043